Natural Cures & Remedies For Beauty!

Natural Remedies To Heal, Boost Metabolism & Keep You Healthy With Ancient Natural Beauty Secrets!

Table Of Contents

Introduction

Instead of relying on chemical substances that are very harmful and unhealthy, you'd soon be carrying out techniques that provide vigor despite being simple, safe, and effective – some merely involve a glass of water. Are you excited? Well, it's no surprise that you are.

If walking gave you a quick energy boost, then jogging (or even running) in place should be a much better option. However, you have to remember that the latter is slightly more tiring than the former – even though jogging in place might be able to give you a temporary boost in energy, doing it for far too long could result in sudden nap times. Usually, a half-a-minute session is more than sufficient.

Thanks for purchasing this book. I hope it will help you boost your energy and remain young and beautiful!

Happy Reading!

Chapter 1: Organic Superfoods

People who lived during the ancient days are considerably known to have a longer lifespan than the people living today. In fact, these ancient people can live up to a hundred years and still remain physically fit and beautiful. Ever wonder why that is? The secret is simple and still true nowadays – they eat nothing but organic super foods.

What are these organic super foods that can help you attain ageless beauty and health? Here are some of them:

1. Salmon

   Common among dieters, Salmon is a super food that can help you attain healthy hair, skin and nails. Aside from being a delicious meal that can keep you full for hours, Salmon is rich in Omega-3 fatty acids, iron, Vitamin B-12 and good fats. 2-3 servings of Salmon can help you get most of your essential fatty acids requirement in a day.

2. Acai Berries and Pomegranates

   These red-colored fruits have anti-oxidant properties which can help protect you from all sorts of diseases, including skin infections. They can also help your skin look younger by fighting off free radicals which causes premature and rapid aging. They likewise promote good blood flow to the skin, making skin regeneration easier and faster.

3. Kiwis, Mangoes and Oranges

High Vitamin C content is the common denominator of all these citrus fruits. Aside from its good taste, these fruits actually help keep your gums and teeth strong. Furthermore, these fruits can help you satisfy your sweet tooth because of its sweet, tangy flavor. No need for you to crave for sugary and unhealthy snacks anymore!

Vitamin C also promotes the production of collagen, a tissue known to improve skin elasticity and texture.

4. Flaxseeds

These little seeds are recommended if you want your skin to be smooth and acne-free! Acne breakouts are oftentimes the result of hormonal imbalance due to lack of proper nutrient supply in the body. Flaxseeds contain high amounts of Omega fatty acids which help balance estrogen levels, thus preventing hormonal imbalance which causes abnormal weight gain, mood swings and acne breakouts.

5. Berries

Feeling bloated and puffy? If so, berries are all you need to get all that extra fluid out of your body! Berries are packed with natural antioxidants, Vitamin C, Potassium and minerals which can help you balance everything in your system, including hormones and excess fluid. With its high antioxidant content, this super food is sure to help you deal with the signs of aging too!

Berries, being a delicious super food can easily be incorporate66d in your meal. You can eat it as a dessert or you can make a smoothie for breakfast. Either way, eating berries would help you remain full longer and curb your sweet tooth.

Who says eating healthy and staying young is difficult? With these super foods, all you have to do is sit back and enjoy delicious yet nutrient-packed snacks!

Chapter 2 – The Best Beverages Selections

Are you a slave to coffee's stimulating power? Are you among those who've already spent a fortune on energy drinks? Maybe you're allergic to caffeine (or any other kind of pick-me-up substance), and that's why you're looking for an alternative. Well, whatever your reason might be, you're about to discover 25 excellent ways to fight tiredness.

Here's the first one – drink a glass of cold water. It's alright if you're a bit skeptical of this suggestion, though. After all, it does seem too simple to provide any noteworthy benefit. However, you should keep in mind that low temperatures have a blood-rushing effect – when cold water passes through the body, the entire circulatory system speeds up its key processes.

So, what happens when blood flows faster (particularly to vital organs)? The body enters a state of alertness (since it's essentially protecting itself from the sudden drop in warmth), which in turn means that the mind would immediately be rid of any thought related to sleep. If you're really running out of energy though, then you might want to rely on a technique that involves sugar.

As you might have expected, the second fatigue-fighting technique is simply drinking a sugar-and-water solution. You're probably thinking of one question right now – isn't sugar a stimulant like caffeine? Truth be told, it isn't – lots of people just assume that it is. After all, kids who eat sweets by the handful cause all sorts of mischief (in other words, they experience periods of hyperactivity).

How does sugar boost alertness then? Well, there are two answers to that. The first one pertains to the sweet granule's energy-rich nature, as well as its structural simplicity. In other words, whenever you drink a sugar-and-water concoction, your body gets an almost immediate increase in energy since it doesn't have to process sugar as much as other vigor-giving substances.

Aside from giving you calories to burn, a sugar-and-water beverage also increases the amount of insulin in your body. To explain a bit further, whenever the body detects that sugar is becoming abundant, it produces more insulin so that sugar levels would go down quickly enough. Insulin has a useful "side effect" though – whenever more of it is available, the brain ends up being stimulated.

If you're not too keen on drinking plain sugar water, then you might want to rely on this tiredness buster – adding lemon juice (or a few slices of the fruit) to a glass of water. Lemon – no matter how sour it is – still contains sugar. It isn't the same as table sugar though, especially since fruit sugar (which experts call fructose) doesn't usually hasten the insulin production process.

Even though lemon water does provide the body with additional energy, it doesn't have as much calories as its table-sugar-containing counterpart. So, is adding fruit juice to H_2O just a poor (but a bit more diabetic-friendly) alternative to mixing sugar and water together? The answer's no. Lemon has an innate sourness that makes it a potent pick-me-up.

After reading that, you might think that drinking extremely sour lemon water is a perfect way of battling sleepiness. That might be a good course of action from time to time, but you shouldn't turn it into a regular habit. If you're wondering why, then you should keep this in mind – anything that's sour can lead to increased gastritis susceptibility and also worsen ulcer-related pain.

Is there a beverage that's suited for someone who doesn't like drinking cold water but has both diabetes and tummy issues? Well, there is – soymilk. It should be pointed out right away though, that the vegan alternative to fresh cow's milk contains moderate amounts of purine – a substance that's linked to both insulin issues and joint concerns.

Simply put, it wouldn't be wise to drink a glass of soymilk every time you feel tired. Drinking a single glass a day should be enough if you have any medical condition that's associated with uric acid. If you're perfectly healthy and you're not getting a lot of purines from the other parts of your diet, then two to three glasses should be fine.

While you're already aware that soymilk isn't something that you should enjoy throughout the entire day, you still don't know how it eliminates the feeling of fatigue. The sheer abundance of Vitamin B12 makes the beverage an excellent alternative to stimulant-containing drinks. That's right; sleepiness is sometimes a sign of Vitamin B12 deficiency.

Is there an alternative to soymilk that's slightly tastier? Even lemon water doesn't taste that great, right? Actually, if you'd add fruits to an ordinary protein shake, then you'd have something that contains both energy-rich carbohydrates and B Vitamins. Since the kind of fruit that you'd add depends on your preferences, you won't have any flavor-related dilemma.

Here's what you must know though – you shouldn't skip the add-on. Even if you're feeling adventurous enough to drink unflavored protein shake (or you simply want to have a lower-calorie beverage), you still need to add a few slices of fruit so that the B Vitamins that you'd get would really be useful. After all, those nutrients mainly hasten the conversion of food to energy.

Just to help you even further, here are several suggestions on which fruits could make your energy-booting beverage much more potent – strawberry (this fruit isn't merely good for the eyes, it's also rich in metabolism-accelerating Vitamin C), banana (a superb, nutritionally-diverse choice for people with digestive issues), and blueberry (known to enhance both mental focus and memory).

Chapter 3 – Activities To Increase Energy

If you like to move a lot, then these exercises should be perfect for you. Yes, physical activity does make your mind more alert, especially since movement prevents thoughts of sleep from popping up.

Here's one kind of exercise that doesn't require too much effort – walking in place. A minute's worth of walking (regardless of how quick your pace is) is often enough to shock the brain into heightening its alertness. What's so good about this simple workout is that you don't even have to move somewhere spacious. You could even do it in front of your desk while you're in the office.

If walking gave you a quick energy boost, then jogging (or even running) in place should be a much better option. However, you have to remember that the latter is slightly more tiring than the former – even though jogging in place might be able to give you a temporary boost in energy, doing it for far too long could result in sudden naptimes. Usually, a half-a-minute session is more than sufficient.

There are instances in which standing up isn't even an option. Well, you shouldn't worry since there are pick-me-up routines that could be done while sitting. Leg lifts are excellent examples of those while-seated exercises. If you're wondering whether it's difficult, then just think about this – the activity simply requires you to lift your legs, one after the other, about twenty times.

While leg lifts are definitely a lot safer than most other

exercises, you still need to follow a few precautionary reminders. For one, you have to check whether your seat is sturdy enough to support your weight (particularly while you move). Aside from that, you mustn't keep your body lifted (with your arms) while raising your legs – even though that seems fun, your shoulders (or the chair) might give out.

If you know for a fact that your body is the very definition of strength, and you're quite confident that your seat wouldn't break even if it isn't used in the normal way, then you might want to try doing body lifts. Just hold on to your chair's armrests and try to lift your entire body upwards. After you've reached the maximum height, move back down slowly.

How many repetitions of that up-and-down movement should you do? There's no specific answer to that, but since you're trying to fight sleepiness and you don't want to feel even more tired, then you shouldn't go past 10 counts. It might even be better if you wouldn't exceed the 15-second mark (especially if you could only lift your body slowly).

If you prefer workouts that are much more engaging and you don't have space-limitation issues, then you might want to try doing some jumping jacks. Simply jump and move your feet apart while you're moving your arms right above your head (your palms should touch one another). Once you land and you're in that feet-apart, hands-together position, jump back into the normal standing stance.

Upright leg curls are superb substitutes to jumping jacks. To benefit from upright leg curling, all you need to do is to stand with your feet apart (bend your knees slightly) and then lift one of your legs behind you. Move that leg back down, and begin to raise the other leg. In short, just repeat the moving-back-down motion for one leg as you transition into lifting the other.

Ten seconds' worth of either jumping jacks or standing leg curls should be sufficient to convince your mind and body that they need to stay alert (and burn more calories to keep you awake). It's vital to remind you though, that you have to stretch before and after doing those exercises no matter how brief they might be. If you don't, then you might experience aches and even suffer from injuries.

Chapter 4 – How To Mentally Boost Your Energy

If you start thinking of things that could make you worry or upset you (the opportunities that you've missed in the past for example), then you must refocus your thoughts towards the positive. Elevated blood pressure and tiredness are linked after all, and the last thing that you'd want to happen is to suffer from stroke or heart attack while trying to stay awake.

As you know by now, beating fatigue is often as easy as keeping the mind occupied and preventing it from thinking about sleep. That's why it's also advantageous to play videogames whenever you feel too tired. It's best to point out though, that some types of videogames are much better "stimulants" than the others.

First-person shooters (titles that essentially give you a gun and let you fire away on all sorts of baddies) and arcade-style racers (games that make you forget about car physics and traffic rules) are two excellent choices. A role-playing game (which usually let you explore a virtual world) would also be a good pick, as long as it offers quick bursts of action.

If you're not interested in videogames and you don't intend to try playing them in the near future, then you might want to go a classic route. In other words, you should challenge someone to 30-second guessing game (or a whole minute if you'd like to take turns). Whether you're the one guessing or you're the "quizmaster", you're bound to feel energized.

Did you say that everyone around you is too serious to play a game? That shouldn't be a problem at all. Instead of trying to convince others to take part in your guess-what challenge, simply strike a conversation. It's almost impossible for your mind to fall asleep (no matter how tired you are) while you're talking to someone, especially if the conversation's about something controversial.

Are you worried that you'd pick a bad topic? Well, these should be interesting to almost anyone – animal testing (a debate between human safety and animal rights), human trafficking (why it still exists despite the fact that society has already changed so much), and the global war on terror (whether it actually protects people or it's merely a way to give governments greater control).

Aside from playing games and engaging in conversations, you could also get a fee pep talk. That doesn't mean that you need to look for a person who's willing to encourage you (verbally). All you have to do is to get a device that has access to the web, and afterwards visit your favorite video-sharing website. Look for the site's search bar, key in "free pep talk", and press enter.

Soon enough, you'd be looking at a results page that's linked to hundreds and even thousands of inspirational videos. If the sheer number of motivational clips is a bit off-putting to you, then you shouldn't close that browser. You just have to make your search much more specific using longer word strings – "free pep talk study", "free pep talk career", and "free pep talk life" are a few good examples.

By the way, these mental stimulation strategies are easier to carry out than most other energy-boosting techniques. Unlike workouts for example, these fatigue-fighting methods don't come with the overexertion downsides. That means that it's unlikely to feel even more tired after doing several mind-focused activities. So, don't be afraid to mix and match what you've discovered in this chapter.

Chapter 5 – Reasons For Your Energy Loss

Right now, you already know various ways to combat sleepiness. This chapter contains five additional techniques that might prove to be much more useful than those already discussed – that is, if you have the option to "change" your environment. After all, tiredness is sometimes triggered by the sleep-inducing nature of certain places.

What kinds of locations make people sleepy? You're thinking about that question, right? Well, warm places tend to make the body feel relaxed, and thus they make it harder to stay awake. Rooms that are dimly lit could also make a person think about slumber since the lack of bright lights simulates nighttime darkness. Silence-filled quarters also intensify the yearning for sleep.

After becoming aware of those facts, you've probably thought about places that could have a stimulating effect on tired minds and bodies. Have you considered the park? Parks that have lots of people tend to have an invigorating impact – particularly due to the sheer amount of things that are happening within such recreational areas (the mind finds it difficult not to observe).

If the park near your place is the very definition of tranquility, then you might want to find another energy-giving spot. If you could go to a room that's covered in warm-colored paint, then you might just be able to beat tiredness. Colors that are usually described as visually intense (such as red) are more than capable of grabbing the mind's attention for long periods.

What's so good about that suggestion is that it highlights the possibility of creating your very own power area. In other words, you could choose one part of your home and make its walls much warmer to the eye (through painting, of course). If you often spend time in the office, then you might want to tell your superior about the benefits of warm colors.

Here's another method of battling tiredness – stay near the air conditioner. As you've read a while back (in the first chapter), low temperatures make the body a lot more active internally. So, if ever you'd choose to sit right beside the AC, your body wouldn't be able to prioritize relaxation; instead, it'd be busy protecting your organs from the cold.

There's no denying that some people really hate low temperatures. If you're among them, then you obviously prefer to go someplace warmer. As mentioned though, warmth has a relaxing effect. So, is there a workaround to that dilemma? There's actually one solution, but it'd only be useful if you live near nature – simply enjoy the sunny outdoors while standing.

Staying upright is a top-notch means of minimizing the sleep-inducing effect of warmth. The abundance of oxygen also keeps the mind alert and much more functional no matter how tired you might be – exhaustion is, in part, a sign of having insufficient amounts of oxygen. The sun keeps you awake as well, since it triggers Vitamin D production (yes, it's an energy-releasing nutrient).

Here's a location-related solution to fatigue that would surely suit you if you're in an urban neighborhood – go to the nearest shopping center. Much like parks, malls and marketplaces are often brimming with activity. Unlike parks though, shopping centers are much noisier – remember silence makes the mind focus on the wonders of slumber.

Aside from having various distracting sounds, those shop-filled places are equipped with bright lights. In short, malls and marketplaces represent the busyness of daytime (even at night), and your mind would never begin to think that it's time to sleep while you're in those establishments – not unless you're really running very low on energy and you've been awake for more than a day.

Chapter 6 —Nutrition

Sometimes there's too much fatigue in your body. Should you use the previous tips if you're at the brink of having a tiredness-induced breakdown? Simply put, you shouldn't – unless you're willing to risk your life just to stay awake (being truly productive is even out of the question). These four remaining strategies should help you avoid that kind of danger.

Here's the first (long-term) defense against sleepiness – eating the right way. Yes, your diet might actually be the reason why you're feeling less energetic as of late, especially if you're not getting the right amount of calories each day. So, the question now is this – what's the easiest way to determine your daily caloric needs? Well, you only have to look for calorie calculators online.

It should be pointed out though, that those web-based apps usually require two important pieces of info (aside from age and exercise level) – weight and height. Once you've identified the caloric sweet spot, you'd have to check your diet. Specifically, you must find out whether what you're eating provides you with enough energy – make adjustments if your diet just doesn't cut it.

While it's essential to monitor your caloric intake, you mustn't forget about one vital rule when it comes to eating – timing is the key. To be a bit more specific, you need to eat a lot during breakfast and go relatively moderate at lunch. It is fine if you're skeptical of that fatigue-fighting suggestion, but you should keep in mind that the digestive system also requires energy to function.

As you might have guessed after reading that, your body begins to feel relaxed (or even lethargic) right after you've enjoyed a big meal since most of your energy stores get burned to fuel the entire digestion process. While that effect might be fine early in the morning, it'd surely have a detrimental impact if it occurs after lunchtime (you should be productive during those hours, right?).

You should also ponder upon the amount of sleep that you've been getting. Teens need at least eight and a half hours of slumber every day. Adults, on the other hand, require less – seven hours is sufficient. It shouldn't be a surprise to you that sleep deprivation leads to much bigger alertness issues. After all, your mind and body wouldn't be able to refresh and regenerate themselves.

If you're not convinced of the importance of sleep (and it's link to mental clarity and attentiveness), then you should think about this fact – in the United States alone, roughly a hundred thousand motor vehicle accidents each year are caused by drowsiness – a key sign of sleep deprivation. By the way, more than a thousand of those accidents lead to fatalities.

What's the 25th long-term sleepiness-busting technique? It's actually exercise. Not the kind that you've read about in the second chapter. This is all about moderately lengthy ones that are done on a regular basis. Brisk walking for half an hour each day is a great example of those fitness-boosting activities. Of course, following a workout video works too.

Why's fitness a vital part of the battle against tiredness? Truth be told, people with the right body-mass index use energy at a much more efficient pace than those classified as either overweight or obese. It's also crucial to note that the mind benefits from sufficient physical activity. Regular exercise is a top-notch way of convincing the brain to grow new cells after all.

Wait a minute. Do you know what the body-mass index is? It's a number that represents how much fat you have right now. In other words, it's a simple way of knowing whether you're fit or not. To determine your BMI, just use one of the many fitness calculators online – don't forget to compare the number that you'd get with the standard values though.

Finally, you've become much more knowledgeable on the matter of exhaustion, and you're aware that both short- and long-term solutions to the problem exist. All in all, you should now be able to stop tiredness in its tracks, as long as you remember that all sorts of things could trigger the problem and knowing the specific cause is crucial to pinpointing the best course of action.

Chapter 7: The Ancient Beauty Secrets

Beauty concerns are universal. They've been and will remain an issue for the human race regardless of any age, gender or era. Can you imagine how people in the past managed to survive these beauty dilemmas?

People who lived in the ancient times have found their own ways to achieve ageless beauty. They were curious, driven and brave enough to experiment with their only resource – nature. Luckily for mankind, nature has all the answers. Take a sneak peek at these ancient beauty secrets!

Beauty tips and tricks come and go; they rise and fall according to the latest beauty trends. However, there are some beauty secrets which stood the test of time. These classic beauty secrets have proven themselves to be more resilient than a beauty hype that everybody forgets after a week and that is simply because they deliver on their promises consistently.

But what's so good about these ancient beauty secrets that would get you dying to try and stick to them for good? Here are some of them:

Ancient beauty solutions are natural

Going back to the past might be helpful when it comes to beauty ideas. The pureness of the materials they use back then (when there was nothing but nature to turn to) is simply too good to forget. There were no harmful chemicals to speak of, only pure natural goodness.

Ancient beauty solutions are raw

Our elders did not care much about product processing. Without the technological breakthroughs during that time, you cannot really expect their beauty products to be as carefully processed as the products sold in the market today. This would only mean one thing – ancient beauty remedies are made from nothing less than raw and roughly processed materials in its purest and most natural state. As such, it retains most of the natural goodness that it contains which would otherwise be stripped off by product processing.

Ancient beauty solutions do not trigger harmful effects

These ancient secrets are made of pure natural goodness which causes little or no harm at all to the body. This would mean fewer health concerns and worry about the things you're putting in your body. By using natural beauty remedies, you can always have the peace of mind knowing that you can get beautiful without compromising your health.

Ancient beauty solutions are usually cheap and even FREE!

Ancient beauty treats are all good news for anyone who wants to get beautiful on a budget. The good thing about these ancient beauty items is that most of them can be found in your backyard or kitchen. They don't always have to be in an expensive salon or spa that you can't afford to go to every single time a pimple or two pops out. All of these lead us to believe in one thing: *you can never put a price on beauty!*

Chapter 8: Stay Beautiful With Essential Oils

Then and now, essential oils have been a beauty staple that never goes out of trend. They are very much used as an ingredient in moisturizers because of its rich, soothing and moisturizing properties. Take a look at some of the essential oils used by people then and now to attain a natural and ageless beauty that shines!

1) Sunflower Oil

   Sunflower oil is derived from sunflower seed extracts which are a rich source of Vitamin E. The benefits of this essential oil have already been recognized around the world and here are some of them:

   a) Lightens scars and unwanted marks on the body

   b) Moisturizes the face, hair and nails

   c) Act as eye moisturizer to lighten eye circles and minimize eye puffing

   d) Soothes skin irritation and insect bites

   e) Act as overall body moisturizer gentle enough even for people with sensitive skin

   f) Serves as make up remover

   With all these benefits at hand, you wouldn't go wrong

with a bottle or two of this miracle oil. The good news is that sunflower is abundant, so its by-products including its oil are sold in the market at affordable prices.

2) Baobab Oil

Baobab Oil is an essential oil derived from the seeds of the Baobab tree. This tree, though may be found in other parts of the world, is native to Africa. In Africa, this oil was first used in the ancient times for the treatment of muscle aches and rheumatism. However, other uses for this oil have been discovered. In Zambia, Africa people used this oil during bath for babies, noting its moisturizing and cleansing property mild enough to take care of sensitive baby skin. Later on, it became a beauty staple used to help maintain skin elasticity and regeneration very much needed to maintain an ageless face.

3) Camellia Oil

To have that ageless beauty, a healthy hair is a must. Remember that it is not only the skin and the face that you should be wary of because hair as the crowning glory can make or break your appearance. The next question is, how do you maintain healthy hair? Camellia Oil can help you in that department!

Camellia Oil is an essential oil used by Japanese women in order to keep their hair sleek and healthy. Camellia Oil has high oleic acids, protein and glycerides content which is perfect for nourishing the hair. The oil is potent enough to allow you to get rid of your usual hot oil treatment. Just put a teaspoon of Camellia Oil to cover your hair, put on a hot towel for 20 to 30 minutes and you're as good as salon-pampered!

4) Tea Tree Oil

Pimples and blemishes are among the most common facial problems that people have nowadays thanks to the polluted environment and chemical-laden products. With all the dirt in the surroundings, it is not surprising that most people find it hard to maintain a clear and smooth face.

Old people have had the same problems and most would tell you they managed it using nothing but Tea Tree Oil. Tea Tree Oil has rich anti-oxidant properties to help the face get rid of dirt and impurities which cause acne breakout. It is also rich in other vitamins to help keep your face smooth, elastic and clean all the time.

5) Chamomile Oil

One of the major causes of premature aging is stress. Inevitable as it is, there are other ways on how to diffuse stress and keep your beauty. One of the ancient ways to do it is through aroma therapy, and undoubtedly Chamomile Oil is the perfect partner for such.

Chamomile Oil has a very relaxing scent which can

help your mind and body release tension. It also has moisturizing properties that can help your skin stay fresh and hydrated. Just put some drops onto your bathtub and watch it work wonders as it relaxes your mind and moisturize your skin.

Grab these must-have natural oils for a beautiful and younger you! These oils are nothing but natural, making them far safer than mineral oil - a harmful chemical that most commercial moisturizers have. Remember that your skin deserves only the best and the purest!

Chapter 9: Cure For Wrinkles

Wrinkles are probably one of the first signs of aging that people hate so much. It doesn't only make your skin crease but it also makes your appearance look less radiant. But don't fret yet! There are easy and effective ways on how to combat wrinkles. Below are some of the natural remedies for wrinkles that you can use:

- Egg white and Lemon Face mask

    How to do it:

    Prepare 1 egg and 1 medium-sized lemon. Separate the egg white from the yolk and set it aside. In the meantime, squeeze half a lemon to get its juice and mix it with the egg white. Mix properly. Put the mixture on your face for 10 – 15 minutes. Rinse it off completely with water.

    Benefits of this face mask:

    Egg whites are known to have wrinkle-fighting properties because of their concentrated protein content. It provides a much needed protein supply for the wrinkled skin to make it look and feel firmer. On the other hand, lemon is very rich in Vitamin C which helps your skin fight off bacteria and skin infections. Together, this face mask combination will help you have firm and smooth skin.

- Olive Oil and Oatmeal Face Mask

  How to do it:

  Prepare 2 teaspoon of olive oil and ½ cup of oatmeal. In a bowl, put in the oatmeal and add the olive oil. Mix and mash the ingredients together until it becomes creamy. If it's not creamy enough to stick, add some more oil.

  Benefits of this face mask:

  Oatmeal is known to be a good source of protein and fiber which can also be beneficial to the skin. It fights off germs to make sure that your skin is clear and it serves as a natural exfoliant to ward off dead skin cells. Meanwhile, olive oil serves as skin moisturizer to protect the skin from being too dry after the exfoliation process.

- Aloe Vera and Rosehip Oil Face Mask

  How to do it:

  Snip one Aloe Vera leaf (if you have it) or get some Aloe Vera essence elsewhere. Rosehip oil is often processed, so you have to get it at a nearby organic beauty store.

  If you're using Aloe Vera leaf, just cut it into 2 and apply the juice directly to your face. Leave it on for 10 minutes and rinse. Afterwards, apply rosehip oil all over your face, leave it on for 10 – 15 minutes and rinse off.

Benefits of this face mask:

Aloe Vera is nature's best cure for minor skin problems like allergy, irritation, acne and blemishes. It cleanses the skin thoroughly and leaves the skin smooth and blemish-free, making it a good primer before applying rosehip oil. Rosehip oil on the other hand, is said to reverse wrinkle formation as it soothes and moisturize the skin, making it one of the most coveted ingredients in the cosmetic industry when it comes to anti-aging products.

Say goodbye to wrinkles with the use of these natural remedies! These natural face masks are easily accessible and affordable so you won't have any reason to put up with those creases.

Chapter 10: Ancient Beauty

To stay beautiful and ageless, people who lived in the old days considered some beauty staples as a must-have. Ever wonder what those things are? Take a peek at some of them!

- Flour Corn (also known as blue corn)

    For hundreds of years, Native American tribes like Hopi, Zuni and Navajo have relied on flour corn not only for food and religious rituals but also for its beauty enhancement properties.

    Blue corn (the other name for flour corn) is coarser than yellow corn and is primarily used for making flour or cornmeal. Aside from that, ground flour corn was also used by natives as a skin cleanser and purifier. It was rubbed to the skin before the start of rituals and ceremonies, on the belief that it could rinse off impurities. It acts as skin exfoliant, ridding the skin of dead skin cells and promoting faster cell regeneration. Because it was easily accessible especially for farmers, people of the tribes always carry a bag or two of this beauty must have.

- Fireweed

    Before contemporary winter coats have been tailored, people back then used animal skin and fireweed to protect their skin from the cold. The root of the fireweed plant is dried, powdered and stored up as a winter must have. The powdered fireweed is rubbed into the skin for protection against the harsh effects of the cold.

- Saw Palmetto

  Back when hormonal imbalance wasn't a common knowledge, native people used Saw Palmetto to get rid of facial hair in women who are experiencing high testosterone levels. As studies now suggest, Saw Palmetto helps regulate excessive hair growth by effectively suppressing DHT production (testosterone derived) in the body.

- Sweet grass

  Considered as sacred, this flat-leafed bladed grass was used to purify both individuals and surroundings. As a beauty regimen though, it was used to treat windburn and dry skin. Some people also boil it to make a tea to be used as hair tonic and body fragrance.

- Wild Mint

  Cheyenne Indians have been using wild mint as hair oil for quite a long time now. Wild mint has anti-inflammatory properties that help the scalp and hair remain itch-free. In addition to that, Thompson Indians also used Wild Mint tonic for hair dressing purposes.

- Yucca

  Baldness and thinning hair are also prominent signs of aging. One of the ways people in the old days handled the same is with the use of Yucca plant. The roots of the Yucca plant were crushed and used as hair wash for balding people and newborns alike to help promote hair growth.

Native people have nothing but nature to rely on when it comes to their beauty needs. However, this didn't stop them from being beautiful with these natural secrets! As modern as today is, it wouldn't hurt to try these ancient secrets, would it?

Chapter 11: Taking Care Of Your Skin

Not contented with your skin? Do you feel like you can have a better skin than what you have? That's perfectly fine because you're ahead of the game. In fact, most people take their skin for granted and just wait for their skin to look old enough before they even bother to care.

A glowing skin can be attained in two ways: by *doing* some things and by *avoiding* others. Listed are the dos and don'ts for a skin that glows!

What to do:

- Relieve stress through aromatherapy

- Go natural and avoid chemical-laden products as much as possible

- Eat healthy

- Exercise for at least 20 minutes a day

- Get ample sleep (at least 6-8 hours of sound and deep sleep)

What *not* to do:

- Smoke cigarettes

- Drink too much liquor

- Sleep with make up on

- Expose yourself to the sun for long periods of time

As much as people should know what they should do, it is sometimes knowing what they should avoid that makes the total difference. Now that you know both, you are now one step closer to your goal!

Chapter 12: New Anti-Aging Solutions

There are beauty secrets that you often hear about while there are some that you never even knew existed. These are uncommon, never-heard-of natural beauty remedies that will surprise you up a bit until you discover the wonders that they can do for your body. Read on to know more about these exotic beauty secrets!

1. Rooibos

   Rooibos is a plant exclusively found in Cape Town, South Africa. The leaves of this plant were made into a red bush tea used both as an anti-allergen and an antioxidant. The essence of the tea has been used to treat skin conditions such as eczema, dermatitis, rashes and inflammation.

2. Pearl Powder

   Pearl powder is an ancient Chinese secret to beautiful skin. It is made of crushed and powdered oyster shells and is known to contain essential amino acids to rejuvenate the skin. More often than not, pearl powder is used together with a mixture of honey and egg yolk so treat inflammation and soothe skin irritations.

3. Cactus

Who knew cactus have anti-aging properties? This prickly pear contains a lot of nutrients such as Riboflavin, B12, Vitamin A and Vitamin D, all known to nourish the skin and halt aging. Overall, it helps increase skin elasticity and speeds up cell regeneration.

4. Persimmon

Want to be as flawless as a geisha? Persimmon might just be the magic you're looking for! This is exactly the Japanese beauty secret dating back in the geisha days. Persimmon is a Japanese fruit containing a lot of vitamins and minerals like phosphorous, magnesium and iodine. Persimmon is often combined with whipped cream before it is applied to the face to help create a flawless complexion.

These exotic beauty ingredients may not be always accessible, but still it's good to know and experiment a little with your beauty regimen from time to time. Go ahead and try some of these exciting beauty recipes when you feel like it!

Chapter 13: Maintain A Youthful Look

Having a youthful glow can be achieved almost instantly with all the cosmetic procedures available nowadays. In fact, you can immediately have a glowing skin right after you did a facial treatment for as short as 15 minutes. However, the real challenge lies in keeping your appearance healthy in the long haul and without much reliance on cosmetic procedures. To be able to do that, you need to build a good beauty regimen to practice over the years. Here are some quick tips on how you could maintain a youthful appearance:

- Brighten up your wardrobe

  Your wardrobe can tell so much about you. It can tell much about your style, preferences, even your age. If your wardrobe consist mostly sweats, pants and boring clothes, it's no wonder that you look way beyond your age. It's now time for you to spice up your wardrobe!

  To look young, you must dress like you are indeed young. The fact that you're getting older doesn't mean that you can't be trendy and stylish. There are so many ways to look younger when you dress up; you just have to be explore a little. For starters, get rid of those plain dark tops and dresses. You can do much better than wear funeral attire. Opt for light colored dresses and do not be all covered up. Show a bit of skin and know what your physical assets are.

- Exfoliate and moisturize

  Sometimes, the skin looks aged because of the dead skin cells lurking around your body. These are old layers of the skin which turns dark and needs to be exfoliated from time to time. You have to know that the body goes through natural exfoliation but the process can take long. As such, it wouldn't hurt for you to help in the natural exfoliating process by using exfoliants such as body scrubs and salts. However, don't forget to moisturize right after exfoliating because your body loses its natural moisture in the process.

  Putting on moisturizer is also a must for young-looking skin. Dry skin tends to patch up easily, making it prone to itch and skin irritations. While the body has natural moisture, factors like sun exposure, stress, and long bath time can take it away, leaving your skin dry. Always bring a moisturizer with you so your skin is sure to stay hydrated all the time!

- Relax once in a while

  Stress is probably one of the main causes of premature aging. While stress is an inevitable part of life, you shouldn't let it get in the way of looking and feeling younger. Give yourself a break and relax those fine lines for a while! This will help your body cope with all the strains and pressure of life. You deserve it!

- Laugh every chance you get

  Laugh lines are surely better than wrinkles. By laughing, you release some of the tension in your body, making you feel lighter and happier. Science would also tell you that smiling uses far less face muscles than frowning, so it helps your facial muscles relax a bit. Most importantly, laughing takes away 10 years off your age by making you look radiant and problem-free!

Being youthful isn't all about being young in age; it's more about being young at heart. Nourish yourself as an individual in all aspects in your life and that youthful appearance will surely follow!

Chapter 14: The Advantages Of Coconut Oil & Honey

Almost every beauty secret makes mention of these two very potent gifts of nature – honey and coconut. Both of them have anti-aging properties which can cure almost every aging problem there is. Continue reading to discover more about these miracle ingredients!

Honey:

Raw honey is known for its antibacterial properties. It keeps the face clean enough to ward off infections, acne breakouts and blemishes. It also has antioxidants which helps fight off free radicals that destroy healthy cells in the body.

Honey is also a good cure for people who are suffering from large pores because of its clarifying properties. Honey goes down to unclog the pores of dirt and grime and leaves the skin clear. Honey can be used directly on the face as mask or you may also combine it with lemon.

Coconut Oil:

Coconut oil on the other hand, is one of nature's most powerful moisturizers. It is also said to protect the skin from the harmful rays of the sun. Coconut oil is mainly composed of saturated fat, Vitamin E and protein which are the essentials for keeping your hair, scalp, skin, nails and body moisturized. This is also one of the safest natural products since very few are reported to have experienced adverse effects to it.

The good news about these natural cures is that they are available almost everywhere. You can drop by any grocery store and find one (at an affordable price too).

Chapter 15: Staying Young & Beautiful

After reading the chapters of this book, you are surely excited to try all of the stuff you read. Fortunately for you, that is the way forward to a younger and healthier you!

However, all the things that you've learned so far still have to be taken under several considerations. You cannot just jump in without knowing certain things. Here are the final considerations that you need to think about before making any changes to your beauty regimen:

- Health concerns/issues

  Your present health condition should be your primary consideration when making any changes on your diet and regimen. Of course, the changes that you will make should suit, or at least be harmless to your health. After all, what good is it if it's going to just make you ill?

  Always seek the advice of your doctor prior to any changes especially if you have a sensitive condition, i.e. pregnant, lactating, etc. This will give you the peace of mind you need.

- Allergic triggers

  The common misconception is that if it's natural, no skin irritation whatsoever can occur. This is completely wrong! Allergic reactions can occur to anyone, no matter how pure and natural the products they use are. For example, some people are naturally allergic to milk (lactose intolerant), mint and shrimp. Because of that, you have to know the contents of what you are putting in your body as well as your allergic triggers. If you have a history of allergic reaction to honey or coconut oil, might as well stop using them even though it has great anti-aging properties. The good news is that there are other alternatives that you may use on your skin. You just have to find what suits you best.

- Time and budget

Time and budget are also considerations that you should take into account. Most of the time, the natural products aren't as easily accessible as the commercial ones so you really have to make an effort in finding them. Just keep in mind that it will be worth it in the end!

- Proper mindset

The last and more important thing is to have the proper mindset. Feeling young and beautiful is not always about having a youthful appearance (although that is important too). Sometimes, you just need to be in the proper state of mind to feel really content and happy about yourself and no amount of makeover can be better than that. Just make sure that whatever you do, you do it because you want to and not because you want to please other people. After all, it is your life and it is you who will make the effort and reap the consequences.

You are now primed and ready to step ten years younger than your age! Go explore and discover all the things life has to offer as you feel more energized, healthier and younger!

Conclusion

Thank you again for purchasing this book.

I am extremely excited to pass this information along to you, and I am so happy that you now have read and can hopefully implement these strategies going forward.

I hope this book was able to help you understand the different ways to pamper your body using natural recipes and how to maintain an ageless beauty throughout the years.

The next step is to get started using this information and to hopefully live a healthy, satisfying and happy life!

Please don't be someone who just reads this information and doesn't apply it, the strategies in this book will only benefit you if you use them!

If you know of anyone else that could benefit from the information presented here please inform them of this book.

Finally, if you enjoyed this book and feel it has added value to your life in any way, please take the time to share your thoughts and post a review on Amazon. It'd be greatly appreciated!

Thank you and good luck!

Legal Notice

Disclaimer Notice

distribution, sale, or any other element of this book responsible for any losses, direct or indirect, which are incurred as a result of the use of information contained within this document, including, but not limited to, -errors, omissions, or inaccuracies. Because of the rate with which conditions change, the author and publisher reserve the right to alter and update the information contained herein on the new conditions whenever they see applicable.

www.ingramcontent.com/pod-product-compliance
Lightning Source LLC
Chambersburg PA
CBHW072018290526
45787CB00013B/1332